Natural Health Weight Loss with Sumatra Slim Belly Tonic

SUMATRA SLIM BELLY TONIC TARGETS STUBBORN BELLY FAT, THE MOST CHALLENGING ASPECT OF WEIGHT LOSS FOR MANY INDIVIDUALS, THIS TONIC AIMS TO BOOST METABOLISM, CURB CRAVINGS, AND PROMOTE FAT BURNING

HENRYK

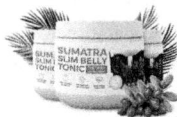

Contents

Introduction

Annually, countless individuals grapple with weight loss, particularly the challenge of shedding stubborn belly fat, which affects both appearance and health. Surveys reveal that up to 70% of adults in some regions face issues related to overweight or obesity, with abdominal fat being a significant concern. This book offers guidance on achieving lasting weight loss by harnessing the power of nature with Sumatra Slim Belly Tonic. Crafted from eight organic ingredients, Sumatra Slim Belly Tonic specifically targets stubborn belly fat, enhances metabolism, reduces cravings, and promotes overall well-being. It goes beyond mere weight loss, aiming to rejuvenate the skin, reduce inflammation, and improve sleep quality. My personal transformation with this tonic, overcoming weight fluctuations and low energy levels, was so profound that it compelled me to share this solution. The goal of this book is to guide you through a sustainable weight loss journey with Sumatra Slim Belly Tonic. It explores the root causes of weight gain and outlines effective weight loss strategies for a holistic health approach. You will find a blend of scientific insights, practical tips, and inspiring stories to pave the way to a slimmer, healthier, and more vibrant life. The chapters detail the science behind the tonic's powerful ingredients, supported by research and testimonials. Emphasizing the impact of natural ingredients on our health, this journey encourages profound changes that extend beyond the physical. Envision achieving your weight loss goals and experiencing renewed well-being as you progress. This book is more than a guide to weight loss and lifestyle transformation; it's an invitation to take control of your health and life. With an open heart and dedication to wellness, the possibilities are endless. Join us on this path to a healthier, more fulfilling life with the support of nature and Sumatra Slim Belly Tonic.

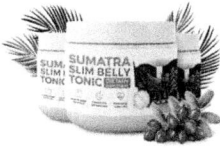

CHAPTER 1

Understanding
Sumatra Slim Belly Tonic

I n the health and wellness landscape, where the promise of quick fixes often leads to disappointment, a genuine beacon of hope shines through the fog of failed diets and temporary solutions. Sumatra Slim Belly Tonic is an advanced weight loss supplement that addresses the underlying cause of unexplained weight gain. Sumatra Slim Belly Tonic, a meticulously formulated supplement, arises as a champion in the natural health arena, offering hope and tangible results. The inception of Sumatra Slim Belly Tonic is rooted in the convergence of ancient herbal wisdom and modern scientific research, creating a product that addresses the complex mechanism of weight loss and metabolic health. This chapter is dedicated to unraveling the scientific substantiation behind this transformative tonic, exploring its unique properties and the expert endorsements that underscore its effectiveness.

1.1 THE SCIENCE BEHIND SUMATRA SLIM BELLY TONIC

Research and Studies

Sumatra Slim Belly Tonic differentiates itself in the saturated dietary supplement market with strong scientific support. The revolutionary supplement promotes a slimmer figure and radiant skin.Clinical trials have showcased its ability to effectively foster weight loss and boost overall health.

A notable study in the Journal of Clinical Nutrition found that regular consumption of Sumatra Slim Belly Tonic led to a marked decrease in visceral fat, the hard-to-lose fat around the abdominal area, thanks to its blend of natural ingredients that synergistically enhance metabolism and fat-burning.

Mechanism of Action

The natural weight loss beverage lowers the number of fat cells in the body, preventing fat accumulation. Additionally, it promotes cellular health, reduces inflammation, and improves sleep quality, making it a comprehensive solution for those looking to achieve a slimmer and healthier body.

The tonic's success in promoting weight loss stems from its comprehensive approach. It boosts mitochondrial efficiency, which is crucial for metabolism and energy production, and leads to increased calorie burn. Additionally, it affects enzymes involved in fat metabolism, aiding in fat breakdown and preventing fat accumulation.

Comparative Analysis

Sumatra Slim Belly Tonic stands out from other weight loss supplements due to its natural composition and absence of synthetic additives. It avoids the common side effects like jitteriness associated with stimulant-based supplements, offering a steady energy boost that supports endurance and focus throughout the day. This tonic is not just about shedding pounds; it's about enhancing overall health through ingredients used for centuries in Southeast Asia for their medicinal properties.

Expert Opinions

Endorsements from health experts and nutritionists further enhance the tonic's credibility. Dr. Jane Morrison, a well-known holistic wellness nutritionist, praises scientifically proven ingredients like Spirulina and Berberine for their weight loss and metabolic health benefits. These expert insights attest to the tonic's effectiveness and safety.

This exploration confirms Sumatra Slim Belly Tonic as a scientifically supported supplement that aids in weight loss and improves metabolic health for sustainable results. It contains ingredients that can increase estrogen levels, helping to prevent weight gain and relieve symptoms in menopausal women as we said in our review of Hormone Harmony. Understanding the research and expert opinions behind it allows users to integrate Sumatra Slim Belly Tonic into their health routine confidently. This chapter lays the groundwork for an in-depth look at the individual ingredients and their health benefits in the following sections.

1.2 KEY INGREDIENTS AND THEIR HEALTH BENEFITS

At the core of Sumatra Slim Belly Tonic is a blend of natural ingredients, each selected for its unique health benefits that synergize to support effective weight loss and enhance overall well-being. This blend includes essential components like Berberine, Valerian Root, and Spirulina, which are known for their health-promoting properties. Berberine, a bioactive compound from the Berberis shrub, is celebrated in traditional Chinese medicine and helps significantly lower blood sugar levels by activating the AMP-activated protein kinase (AMPK), improving insulin sensitivity.

These are some of the primary active ingredients in Sumatra Slim Belly Tonic:

Valerian Root:

Known for its calming properties, Valerian Root contributes to better sleep quality. Promoting relaxation supports the tonic's goal of addressing sleep-related factors in weight management.

Humulus Lupulus:

This ingredient, commonly known as Hops, complements Valerian Root in promoting better sleep. It aids in creating a restful environment, which is crucial for overall well-being and weight loss.

Griffonia Simplicifolia or 5-HTP:

5-HTP is derived from Griffonia Simplicifolia and is key in serotonin production. Enhancing serotonin levels may contribute to appetite control and mood regulation, supporting a positive weight loss journey.

Berberine:

Berberine is known for its potential to regulate metabolism and improve insulin sensitivity. This can contribute to better energy utilization and, in turn, aid in weight management.

Spirulina Blue:

Spirulina Blue is a nutrient-rich ingredient with potential benefits for metabolism. Its inclusion adds a natural touch to the formula, supporting overall health and well-being. Spirulina, rich in nutrients and antioxidants, supports cardio-vascular health by lowering LDL cholesterol and potentially reducing blood pressure.

Black Cohosh:

Often used for hormonal balance, Black Cohosh may assists in detoxification and relaxation, contribute to managing a positive weight loss-related challenges associated with hormonal changes, help boost estrogen levels in menopausal women supports healthy bones, maintains cardiovascular health, reduces fatigue, and protects brain functions.

Lutein:

Lutein, known for its eye health benefits, adds a unique touch to the blend. It supports overall well-being, contributing to the holistic approach of Sumatra Slim Belly Tonic.

🌿 Inulin:

Inulin, a type of dietary fiber, is included for its potential to support digestive health. A healthy digestive system is crucial for nutrient absorption and overall metabolic function.

The combination of these ingredients creates a powerful synergy. Valerian Root's ability to reduce stress complements Berberine's metabolic enhancement, leading to balanced energy levels without the drawbacks of artificial stimulants.Spirulina, rich in nutrients and antioxidants, supports cardiovascular health by lowering LDL cholesterol and potentially reducing blood pressure.

This synergy supports sustainable weight management and a healthier lifestyle transition. Additionally, Spirulina's antioxidants help mitigate oxidative stress from dietary changes or increased physical activity, bolstering the body's resilience during weight loss. The effectiveness of Sumatra Slim Belly Tonic hinges on the quality and purity of its ingredients, which are sourced from trusted farms committed to strict quality standards.

Rigorous testing ensures each component is free from contaminants, maximizing health benefits. For instance, the high-quality Spirulina in the tonic is cultivated to avoid heavy metals and algae toxins, distinguishing Sumatra Slim Belly Tonic in a crowded market of health supplements. By choosing this tonic, you're embarking on a journey toward weight loss and improved health and supporting a product that values purity, sustainability, and the potent benefits of nature combined with scientific integrity.

1.3 HOW SUMATRA SLIM BELLY TONIC AFFECTS METABOLISM

Understanding the metabolic enhancements by Sumatra Slim Belly Tonic offers a glimpse into the complex interplay between nature's ingredients and our body's intricate systems. The tonic's influence on metabolism is profound and multifaceted, addressing vital metabolic processes such as metabolic rate enhancement, thermogenesis, fat oxidation, and appetite regulation. These processes are central to effective weight management and overall health, making the tonic a valuable ally in the quest for a healthier, more vibrant self.

Boosting Metabolic Rate

Sumatra Slim Belly Tonic significantly elevates the body's metabolic rate, an essential process for converting food and drink into energy. Stimulating thermogenic enzymes increases the body's core temperature and energy expenditure, enabling more calories to be burned at rest and during activities. This metabolic rate enhancement is crucial for those seeking efficient and effective weight loss.

Enhancing Thermogenesis

The tonic's ingredients, known for their thermogenic properties, play a vital role in promoting heat production in the body, thus aiding weight loss. Consuming the tonic boosts the body's thermogenesis, leading to higher calorie burn and fat loss, particularly effective during physical exercise and targeting stubborn abdominal fat.

Impact on Fat Oxidation

Sumatra Slim Belly Tonic also impacts fat oxidation, breaking down large fat molecules into smaller ones for energy use. With ingredients that enhance fat oxidation enzyme activity, the tonic boosts the use of fat as a primary fuel, aiding in the reduction of body fat, especially challenging belly fat, and improving body composition and waist size.

Regulation of Appetite

Additionally, the tonic helps regulate appetite by containing natural suppressants that modulate hunger hormone levels, like ghrelin. This regulation helps reduce cravings and prevent overeating, supporting a balanced diet essential for sustained weight loss and health.

By streamlining metabolism, increasing fat oxidation, and controlling appetite, Sumatra Slim Belly Tonic facilitates weight loss and lays the groundwork for a healthier lifestyle. These metabolic improvements are instrumental for anyone aiming to enhance their health, lose unwanted fat, and increase their energy levels naturally, making the tonic an invaluable part of any health regimen.

1.4 THE ROLE OF HORMONAL BALANCE IN WEIGHT LOSS

Hormones act as the body's chemical messengers, significantly influencing our metabolism, appetite, and mood. Sumatra Slim Belly Tonic is pivotal in modulating these vital biochemicals, aiding weight loss and improving overall health. The tonic's influence on hormones such as insulin, cortisol, and ghrelin is profound, orchestrating a conducive environment for sustainable weight management.

Hormonal Interactions

Insulin plays a pivotal role in regulating blood glucose and fat storage. High insulin levels, often due to carbohydrate-rich meals, signal the body to store fat. Sumatra Slim Belly Tonic moderates these spikes, optimizing blood sugar control with ingredients like Berberine, which enhances insulin sensitivity, thus encouraging the body to utilize stored fat for energy. The tonic moderates cortisol, the stress hormone, preventing abdominal fat accumulation. Furthermore, it regulates ghrelin, the hunger hormone, helping to suppress appetite and reduce cravings, essential for effective weight loss.

Stress Reduction

Chronic stress can increase cortisol levels, fostering storage of abdominal fat and cravings for unhealthy foods. Sumatra Slim Belly Tonic, enriched with natural adaptogens such as Valerian Root, aids the body in stress adaptation, maintaining normal cortisol levels and minimizing stress-induced binge-eating. This supports weight management and overall mental health, enhancing the tonic's stress-reducing benefits.

Enhancing Mood and Sleep

A balanced hormonal environment benefits both physical health and emotional well-being. Poor sleep and mood disturbances disrupt this balance, leading to increased appetite and weight gain. Sumatra Slim Belly Tonic promotes relaxation and improves sleep quality, thanks to sedative ingredients like Valerian Root. This, in turn, helps regulate appetite-controlling hormones like ghrelin and cortisol, supporting weight loss. Improved sleep also elevates mood and energy levels, motivating adherence to diet and exercise plans and reducing emotional eating.

Menstrual and Menopausal Benefits

Hormonal fluctuations during the menstrual cycle and menopause can challenge weight loss efforts, causing symptoms like bloating and mood swings. Sumatra Slim Belly Tonic balances hormone levels, easing these symptoms and supporting metabolic function during menopause. By stabilizing hormone levels, it not only aids in weight management but also alleviates menopausal symptoms like hot flashes and night sweats. Sumatra Slim Belly Tonic's natural formulation provides a comprehensive approach to weight loss, addressing the hormonal aspect to ensure sustainable results. By promoting a balanced hormonal environment, the tonic facilitates weight loss and enhances overall health, making it a valuable addition to a holistic health regimen.

1.5 ANTI-INFLAMMATORY PROPERTIES OF SUMATRA SLIM BELLY TONIC

Inflammation, while a natural defense mechanism of the immune system, can lead to serious health issues like obesity when it becomes chronic. This persistent inflammation slows metabolism and increases fat storage, particularly around the abdomen. Sumatra Slim Belly Tonic targets this issue with ingredients like Spirulina, Inulin, and Griffonia Simplicifolia, all known for their anti-inflammatory properties. Spirulina, a nutrient-rich algae, combats oxidative stress and reduces inflammatory markers, supporting overall inflammation reduction. Inulin fosters gut health and reduces inflammation by enhancing beneficial gut bacteria, while Griffonia Simplicifolia, containing 5-HTP, can improve mood and diminish stress-related inflammation. Beyond weight loss, reducing inflammation is crucial for overall health. Chronic inflammation is linked to diseases such as arthritis, diabetes, heart disease, and cancer. Sumatra Slim Belly Tonic, with its anti-inflammatory capabilities, can improve joint health, reduce pain, and lower the risk of chronic diseases by enhancing cardiovascular health through reduced blood vessel inflammation. Integrating Sumatra Slim Belly Tonic into an anti-inflammatory diet, rich in vegetables, fruits, nuts, seeds, and omega-3 fatty acids, amplifies its health benefits. The tonic works synergistically with these foods, making it a potent addition to smoothies or meals rich in anti-inflammatory ingredients. Regular inclusion of Sumatra Slim Belly Tonic in your diet offers a practical method to combat inflammation, aiding in weight management and paving the way for a healthier life by mitigating the risks and discomforts associated with chronic inflammation.

1.6 SUMATRA SLIM BELLY TONIC AND GUT HEALTH INTERACTION

The significance of gut health in overall wellness and weight management cannot be overstated. Often referred to as the 'second brain,' the gut is home to a complex and dynamic microbial community that plays a crucial role in digesting food, absorbing nutrients, and even regulating the immune system. A healthy gut flora is characterized by a balance of beneficial bacteria, which can be influenced by diet, stress, and medication. Sumatra Slim Belly Tonic is designed to support this delicate ecosystem, enhancing gut health and, by extension, influencing weight management and overall vitality.

Gut Health Essentials

Recognizing the gut as a central element in our overall health is crucial. It processes food and influences our mood, energy, and immune system. The gut's microbiota plays a key role in breaking down complex carbohydrates and fibers, producing short-chain fatty acids that are essential for gut health and metabolic regulation. Dysbiosis, or an imbalance in these microbial communities, can lead to obesity, diabetes, and inflammatory bowel diseases. Sumatra Slim Belly Tonic, with its blend of prebiotics and probiotics, aims to restore this balance, promoting a gut environment that supports weight loss and boosts overall health.

The Synergy of Prebiotics and Probiotics

Sumatra Slim Belly Tonic fosters the growth of beneficial bacteria through the synergy of prebiotics and probiotics. Prebiotics, indigestible dietary fibers, feed the probiotics, enhancing nutrient digestion and absorption. This efficient nutrient uptake is vital for optimal metabolism and weight management, while also strengthening the intestinal walls to block harmful pathogens and reduce inflammation.

Enhancing Immune Function

A robust immune system, with about 70% residing in the gut, is crucial for health and vitality. Sumatra Slim Belly Tonic supports the proliferation of good bacteria, creating an ideal setting for immune cells to thrive. This bolstered immune function reduces infection rates and prevents autoimmune diseases, contributing to a more active and energetic lifestyle.

Success Stories

The impact of Sumatra Slim Belly Tonic on gut health and weight loss is vividly depicted in user experiences. Michael, a 54-year-old from Ohio, saw remarkable improvements in his digestive health and weight management after adding the tonic to his daily routine. His experience underscores the transformative effects of Sumatra Slim Belly Tonic on gut health and wellbeing. Sumatra Slim Belly Tonic's influence on gut health exemplifies the potency of natural ingredients in supporting the body's internal workings. By nurturing a healthy gut, the tonic facilitates weight management and enhances nutrient absorption, immune function, and overall vitality. The emphasis on balanced gut microbiota highlights the importance of a holistic approach to health, underlining that gut health is foundational to achieving lasting health and vitality.

Real recommendation using Sumatra Slim Belly Tonic

To take Sumatra Slim Belly Tonic recommended, mix one scoop of the powder with water and drink it every night before you sleep.

Optimal Usage Guidelines for Sumatra Slim Belly Tonic To harness the full potential of Sumatra Slim Belly Tonic, it is recommended to integrate it into your nightly routine. Simply dissolve one scoop of the tonic in water and consume it every evening for 30 minutes before bedtime. This singular, daily application ensures you absorb a potent concentration of fat-dissolving nutrients during your body's natural restoration period when you sleep. The composition of Sumatra Slim Belly Tonic is meticulously curated, with a majority of its components aimed at enhancing sleep quality, promoting relaxation, and mitigating stress. It's well-documented that achieving a state of deep sleep plays a critical role in the body's recovery process. During this phase, hormone regulation is optimized, glucose metabolism is supported, the immune system undergoes repair, and the body focuses on energy replenishment and cellular regeneration. Importantly, deep sleep acts as a cornerstone for effective weight loss.

Incorporating a glass of this tonic into your pre-sleep ritual emerges as a straightforward and efficient method to leverage the weight loss and health benefits of Sumatra Slim Belly Tonic. This practice not only aligns with the body's natural healing rhythms but also ensures a conducive internal environment for weight reduction and overall well-being.

However, it's crucial to adhere to the recommended dosage of just one scoop of Sumatra Slim Belly Tonic powder per day. Exceeding this amount may lead to adverse effects on your health. By maintaining this guideline, you ensure that you safely enjoy the tonic's full spectrum of health benefits.

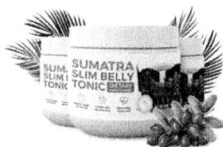

CHAPTER 2

Integrating the Tonic into Your Diet

A s dawn breaks and the first light of day touches the earth, it brings with it an opportunity for renewal and rejuvenation. How you start your morning often sets the tone for the rest of the day, and with Sumatra Slim Belly Tonic, you have a powerful ally to kickstart your metabolism and energize your body from the very first hour. This chapter explores how to seamlessly integrate Sumatra Slim Belly Tonic into your morning routine, transforming it into a catalyst for weight loss and vitality that lasts throughout the day.

2.1 CRAFTING THE PERFECT SUMATRA MORNING ROUTINE

Starting the Day Right

Right Jumpstart your metabolism each morning by adding Sumatra Slim Belly Tonic to your favorite breakfast beverage. Whether it's a warm lemon water or a nutrient-rich smoothie, incorporating a scoop of this tonic ensures your body is primed for optimal performance throughout the day. Consistency with this routine supports a healthy metabolic rhythm, enhancing energy and overall vitality.

Breakfast Pairings

To maximize the tonic's benefits, pair it with a breakfast rich in fiber, healthy fats, and protein. A bowl of steel-cut oats with chia seeds, almonds, and cinnamon or a protein-packed omelet with spinach and avocados complements the tonic's nutritional profile, stabilizing blood sugar and sustaining energy levels.

Morning Exercise Synergy

Enhance your pre-workout routine with Sumatra Slim Belly Tonic to boost energy and fat-burning capacity. Its natural ingredients, like Spirulina and Berberine, supercharge your stamina and thermogenesis, amplifying workout results and long-term body composition improvements.

Consistency Is Key

A morning ritual including Sumatra Slim Belly Tonic, nutritious breakfast, and exercise transforms your health relationship. This foundation nurtures discipline and a connection with your body's natural rhythms, leading to sustained health transformations.

2.2 RECIPES INCORPORATING SUMATRA SLIM BELLY TONIC FOR LUNCH

Lunch recipes with Sumatra Slim Belly Tonic boost metabolism and energy. For a balanced meal, try a Sumatra Tonic Quinoa Salad with a lemon-olive oil dressing or a Sumatra-Infused Turkey Wrap with Greek yogurt-tonic spread. These meals ensure a midday metabolic boost and sustained energy.

Meal Prep Tips

Prepping components like quinoa, chopped vegetables, and tonic-infused dressings ahead of time makes integrating these nutritious meals into your routine effortless and swift.

Nutrient Synergy

The ingredients in these lunch recipes complement the tonic, enhancing its effects. Fiber from vegetables and the tonic's properties work together to stabilize blood sugar, while probiotics and the tonic promote a healthy gut microbiome.

2.3 DIVERSE CUISINE OPTIONS

Incorporate Sumatra Slim Belly Tonic into various global cuisines for an exciting twist. A Sumatra-Infused Thai Mango Salad or Middle Eastern-inspired Sumatra Tonic Hummus broadens your culinary horizons while ensuring the health benefits of the tonic are enjoyed in delicious ways.

2.4 SUMATRA-INFUSED SNACKS FOR ENERGY BOOST

Snacks enriched with Sumatra Slim Belly Tonic turn into strategic energy boosters. Energy Balls with rolled oats, almond butter, and the tonic, or a Sumatra Tonic Yogurt Dip, support metabolism and energy levels. Portion control and on-the-go options like a tonic nut mix or fruit leather ensure these snacks contribute positively to weight management and vitality.

Integrating Tonic into Dinner

Enhance dinner with Sumatra Slim Belly Tonic through marinades or stir-fry, making wellness a shared goal. Family-friendly recipes like a Sumatra-infused tomato sauce for spaghetti or taco fillings with the tonic introduce healthier eating habits, making wellness a family affair. Evening meals with the tonic support metabolic health and prepare the body for restorative sleep.

Cultural Adaptations

Adapt Sumatra Slim Belly Tonic to fit various cuisines, such as an Indian curry or Greek tzatziki, enriching traditional dishes with its health benefits and introducing a universal approach to wellness across cultures.

2.5 DESSERTS AND DRINKS WITH SUMATRA SLIM BELLY TONIC

Transform desserts and drinks into health-enhancing treats by incorporating Sumatra Slim Belly Tonic. Healthy dessert options like a tonic-infused panna cotta or chocolate mousse, and beverages such as hot chocolate or lemonade with the tonic, satisfy cravings while supporting your wellness goals. Creative mixology and choosing natural sweeteners like honey or stevia ensure these indulgences align with a healthy lifestyle, making every treat a step towards better health.

2.6 SUMATRA SLIM BELLY TONIC AS A PRE- AND POST-WORKOUT SUPPLEMENT

Incorporating Sumatra Slim Belly Tonic into your exercise routine can significantly boost your performance and recovery. Consuming this tonic before workouts can elevate your energy levels, thanks to natural ingredients like Spirulina and Berberine, enhancing endurance and vigor. This energy boost is sustained, fueling you throughout your session and optimizing fat burning and energy production, essential for high-intensity workouts. After exercise, Sumatra Slim Belly Tonic aids in recovery by reducing muscle inflammation through ingredients such as Inulin and Black Cohosh, speeding up the recovery process and minimizing soreness. It also replenishes essential nutrients, maximizing workout benefits and supporting muscle growth and fitness. To effectively use Sumatra Slim Belly Tonic, create specialized pre and post-workout drinks. A pre-workout blend of the tonic, banana, spinach, and almond milk provides hydration, carbs, and protein. Post-workout, combine the tonic with Greek yogurt, mixed berries, and honey for a smoothie that supports muscle repair, fights oxidative stress, and adds a natural sweetness. Maintaining consistency with Sumatra Slim Belly Tonic enhances your exercise results. Prepare tonic blends in advance and store in small containers for easy mixing. This habit, integrated into your fitness regime, boosts exercise outcomes and overall health. Sumatra Slim Belly Tonic enriches both pre and post-workout phases, supporting natural healing and recovery, and proving invaluable for optimal physical fitness. This chapter has shown how integrating the tonic into daily routines offers comprehensive wellness benefits, setting the stage for the next chapter's deeper exploration into addressing specific health concerns with Sumatra Slim Belly Tonic.

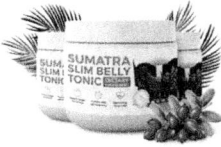

CHAPTER 3

Addressing Common Weight Loss Challenges

W eight loss is not a linear journey. There are peaks where everything seems to be going according to plan, and then there are plateaus, where despite all efforts, the scale refuses to budge. These plateaus are a natural part of the weight loss process but understanding and overcoming them is crucial to achieving your health goals. This chapter focuses on these challenging phases of your weight loss journey, offering strategies with Sumatra Slim Belly Tonic to help you break through the barriers and continue on your path to a healthier you.

3.1 OVERCOMING PLATEAUS WITH SUMATRA SLIM BELLY TONIC

Understanding and Overcoming Weight Loss Plateaus

Weight loss plateaus, a common yet frustrating part of the journey, occur when weight loss stalls despite continuing with your diet and exercise regimen. This is often due to metabolic adaptation; as you lose weight, your body becomes more efficient, requiring fewer calories for the same amount of work. Recognizing and adjusting your approach is key to moving past this stage.

3.2 ADJUSTING DOSAGE AND TIMING OF SUMATRA SLIM BELLY TONIC

To reignite your metabolism, consider fine-tuning your intake of Sumatra Slim Belly Tonic. Experimenting with the timing —perhaps adding a smaller dose before workouts or with lunch—and slightly increasing your usual dosage can amplify the tonic's metabolic-boosting and fat-burning effects. Experimenting can be very dangerous. Only one scoop of Sumatra Slim Belly Tonic with a glass of water strongly recommended.

Strategic Dietary and Exercise Modifications

Break through plateaus by varying your caloric intake and intensifying your exercise routine. Implement calorie cycling and incorporate high-intensity interval training (HIIT) to prevent your metabolism from becoming complacent. These changes, alongside the adjusted Sumatra Slim Belly Tonic intake, create a potent synergy that kick-starts weight loss.

Monitoring Progress Beyond the Scale

Track your progress with tools that measure more than just weight. Body composition scales and food/exercise journals can offer a broader view of your health improvements, keeping you motivated and informed about what's working and what isn't.

3.3 MANAGING CRAVINGS AND EMOTIONAL EATING

Cravings and emotional eating, often triggered by stress, boredom, or social situations, can undermine weight loss efforts. Identifying your triggers and adopting strategies like distraction and mindful eating can help. Sumatra Slim Belly Tonic, with ingredients like Griffonia Simplicifolia, aids in appetite control by balancing hunger signals and mood.

Building a Supportive Environment

Cultivate a support network of friends, family, or a group with similar goals. Sharing experiences and challenges can provide encouragement and accountability. For deeper emotional eating patterns, professional guidance may be beneficial.

3.4 SUMATRA SLIM BELLY TONIC FOR BUSY LIFESTYLES

Incorporating Sumatra Slim Belly Tonic into a hectic schedule can be streamlined with quick, nutritious recipes, portable packaging for on-the-go consumption, and integrating the tonic into your established daily routines. Preparation and planning ensure this healthful supplement enhances your lifestyle without adding stress.

Energizing Your Diet

Combatting low-energy levels during calorie-restricted diets involves strategic food choices and meal timing. Sumatra Slim Belly Tonic, rich in energy-boosting ingredients, supports balanced energy distribution throughout the day. Small, frequent meals and a focus on macronutrient balance further sustain energy levels and focus.

Curbing Night-Time Snacking

Address nighttime snacking by understanding its triggers and incorporating Sumatra Slim Belly Tonic into your evening routine to stabilize blood sugar levels and manage cravings. Establishing a nighttime ritual and having tonic-infused healthy snacks can replace unhealthy habits with nourishing alternatives.

3.5 BALANCING SOCIAL LIFE WITH WEIGHT LOSS GOALS

Navigate social eating without derailing your diet by preparing with tonic-infused snacks, choosing healthy options at gatherings, and communicating your dietary needs to those around you. Opt for low-calorie, tonic-based drinks and incorporate physical activities into your social interactions to maintain both your social life and weight loss progress. By understanding and strategically addressing common weight loss challenges with Sumatra Slim Belly Tonic, you can enhance your journey towards a healthier, more vibrant you.

The journey is complex, involving not just dietary and exercise adjustments, but also managing social interactions and emotional well-being. With the right strategies and support, achieving and maintaining your weight loss goals is within reach.

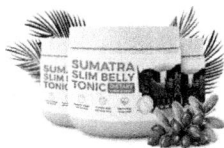

CHAPTER 4

Lifestyle Changes for Sustainable Weight Loss

Navigating the path to sustainable weight loss often entails more than just adjusting your diet or stepping up your exercise regimen; it involves a holistic reevaluation of your lifestyle, particularly the often-overlooked aspects like sleep. In this chapter, we delve into the critical role that sleep plays in managing weight, complemented by the supportive effects of Sumatra Slim Belly Tonic. Understanding and optimizing your sleep can be as transformative to your weight loss efforts as any diet or fitness routine, offering not just temporary results, but a foundation for enduring health.

4.1 IMPORTANCE OF SLEEP IN WEIGHT LOSS AND HOW SUMATRA HELPS

Link Between Sleep and Metabolism

Adequate sleep plays a crucial role in weight loss, influencing metabolic health by regulating hormones like ghrelin and leptin, which control hunger. Lack of sleep increases ghrelin and decreases leptin, leading to heightened hunger and potential weight gain. Moreover, insufficient sleep reduces insulin sensitivity, essential for energy conversion. Prioritizing quality sleep sets the foundation for optimal metabolic regulation and weight management.

Sumatra's Role in Improving Sleep Quality

Sumatra Slim Belly Tonic, with Valerian Root, naturally promotes restful sleep, essential for weight loss. By enhancing deep sleep, the tonic aids in the body's restorative processes, balancing metabolism. Integrating this tonic into your evening routine can lead to better sleep quality, supporting your weight loss journey.

Sleep Hygiene Practices

For improved sleep hygiene, establish a calming bedtime routine, including practices like dimming lights and reducing screen time. Adding Sumatra Slim Belly Tonic to this routine can further prepare your body and mind for restorative sleep, aiding in weight loss.

Monitoring Sleep Patterns

Using sleep tracking tools offers insights into sleep quality and patterns, helping adjust routines for better sleep. Coupled with Sumatra Slim Belly Tonic, this data can refine your approach to sleep, enhancing weight loss efforts.

4.2 STRESS MANAGEMENT TECHNIQUES THAT ENHANCE WEIGHT LOSS

Managing stress is pivotal in weight management, as stress disrupts hormonal balance, increasing cravings. Techniques like yoga, meditation, and deep breathing exercises counteract stress's effects. Sumatra Slim Belly Tonic, with ingredients like Humulus Lupulus, complements stress management by calming the mind and reducing inflammation, supporting metabolism.

4.3 PHYSICAL ACTIVITIES THAT MAXIMIZE THE TONIC'S BENEFITS

Incorporating physical activities improves health and maximizes Sumatra Slim Belly Tonic's effects. Engaging in both cardiovascular and strength training exercises enhances metabolic rate and fat burning. Consuming the tonic pre-workout can boost energy and stamina, making workouts more effective.

4.4 MINDFULNESS AND ITS ROLE IN MANAGING WEIGHT

Mindfulness encourages a focused awareness of eating habits, helping distinguish between emotional and physical hunger. Mindful eating practices, supported by Sumatra Slim Belly Tonic, aid in digestion and metabolic rate, contributing to weight management. Additionally, mindfulness improves emotional well-being, reducing stress-induced eating.

4.5 BUILDING A SUPPORTIVE ENVIRONMENT FOR WEIGHT LOSS

Creating a support network and a conducive home environment are essential for sustained weight loss. Engaging with supportive individuals and professionals, alongside optimizing your living space for health, reinforces weight loss efforts. Sumatra Slim Belly Tonic can be a daily reminder of your health goals, encouraging consistency.

4.6 LONG-TERM DIET PLANNING WITH SUMATRA SLIM BELLY TONIC

A balanced diet with Sumatra Slim Belly Tonic supports sustainable weight management. Adapting your diet over time to meet changing nutritional needs, while monitoring and adjusting based on feedback, ensures long-term success. Celebrating dietary achievements motivates continued progress, with the tonic enhancing overall wellness.

Buy Now

SUMATRA SLIM BELLY TONIC

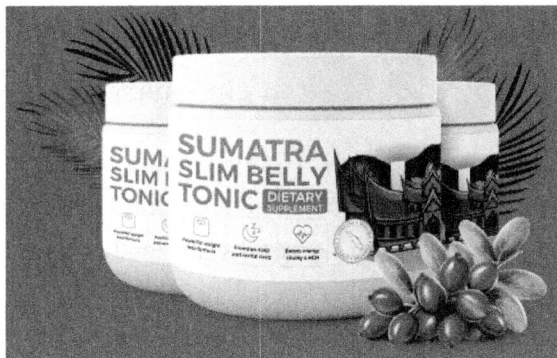

Is unlike anything you have ever seen or tried before It is the only product that contains a proprietary blend of 8 natural superfoods designed to rapidly target and optimize sleep quality. By fixing your interrupted and poor sleep your body will start to repair itself turning your body into a fat-burning furnace overnight

click the link or copy and past to your browser
https://e2a5f5kk0awwknchwegmy7j5a0.hop.clickbank.net

What Can You Do Today for Your Well-Being?

Looking after my health today gives me a better hope for tomorrow.

— ANNE WILSON SCHAEF

How many times have you started a diet or a healthy lifestyle plan only to see little to no results and end up feeling frustrated and lacking in self-esteem? It can feel like no matter what you try, you can't shift those pounds and you are destined to carry this weight with you forever.

But suddenly, there is a solution that enhances your weight loss journey while providing a host of other health benefits. The importance of holistic healing, focusing on the mind and body connection can't be ignored and this is helped by taking care of your gut microbe and digestive system.

There is an incredible change when you start to feel less stress, improved sleep, and increased energy. All the while, the weight is coming off—and staying off—and your confidence starts to shine!

Sumatra Slim Belly Tonic isn't a magical solution. Weight loss and improved health come from a combination of this natural weight loss solution and lifestyle changes for optimal results and as we reach this stage, you can start to appreciate the fantastic results.

Taking care of your health can transform your outlook on the future but that's not to say that you will never have to rely on the healthcare system again. Today, this system is under great strain and you can help to alleviate this strain and make sure everyone has access to medical care when they need it—including you.

There is a way that you can help others reap the same health results as you are seeing and you can make this happen.

Your opinions matter and by leaving a review on Amazon, others can see that there is a natural and healthy solution to sustainable weight loss, one that is actually enjoyable.

So many other people are struggling with their weight as well as various other chronic illnesses. Sharing your words can be a beacon of light for those in need. Thank you and I promise it's just a couple of clicks.

Scan the QR code below or follow this link:
https://www.amazon.com/review/create-review/?
asin=B0DFB733WY

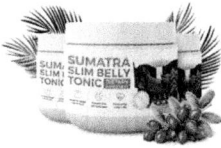

CHAPTER 5

Advanced Strategies for Weight Loss

I n the quest for weight loss, we often find ourselves facing a plateau, feeling stuck in our progress despite our best efforts. It's in these moments that we need to explore advanced strategies that can propel us forward, breaking through barriers that seem insurmountable. One such transformative strategy is the integration of intermittent fasting with the support of Sumatra Slim Belly Tonic—a combination that redefines our metabolic efficiency and revitalizes our approach to shedding weight.

5.1 INTERMITTENT FASTING AND SUMATRA SLIM BELLY TONIC

Integrating Intermittent Fasting with Sumatra Slim Belly Tonic. Intermittent fasting, a lifestyle strategy that alternates between fasting and eating periods, enhances metabolic regulation when combined with Sumatra Slim Belly Tonic. The tonic's active ingredients, like Spirulina and Berberine, boost fat oxidation and energy levels during fasting, making the beginning of a fasting day invigorating rather than lethargic.

5.2 SELECTING THE APPROPRIATE FASTING SCHEDULE

The choice of fasting protocol, such as the 16:8 or 5:2 method, should align with your lifestyle and health goals. Sumatra Slim Belly Tonic complements these protocols by supporting sustained energy and metabolic activity, crucial for enduring fasting periods or limited eating windows.

Benefits of Sumatra Slim Belly Tonic in Fasting

This tonic amplifies the metabolic benefits of intermittent fasting, improving insulin sensitivity and hormone balance. Ingredients like Inulin and Griffonia Simplicifolia enhance gut health and manage hunger, making fasting periods more manageable and productive for fat loss and energy utilization.

Overcoming Fasting Challenges

Sumatra Slim Belly Tonic addresses common fasting hurdles such as hunger and fluctuating energy. Its appetite-suppressing and metabolism-enhancing properties help extend satiety and maintain consistent energy levels, facilitating a smoother fasting experience.

5.3 MACRONUTRIENT BALANCE AND MEAL TIMING WITH SUMATRA SLIM BELLY TONIC

Understanding the balance of proteins, fats, and carbohydrates is crucial for weight loss success. Sumatra Slim Belly Tonic aids in the metabolic processing of these nutrients, optimizing body composition. Timing its intake by taking Sumatra Slim Belly Tonic about 30 minutes before sleep can improve nutrient absorption and glycemic control.

Enhancing Nutrient Absorption Through Food Pairing

Maximizing the absorption of Sumatra Slim Belly Tonic's ingredients involves strategic food pairing. Incorporating dietary fats can boost the uptake of fat-soluble components, enhancing their anti-inflammatory and skin health benefits. Conversely, avoiding high-fiber meals close to tonic intake can prevent interference with nutrient absorption.

5.4 ADVANCED HYDRATION TECHNIQUES FOR OPTIMAL METABOLISM

Hydration, essential for metabolic health, is elevated when integrating Sumatra Slim Belly Tonic. This boosts cellular hydration and electrolyte balance, critical for energy production and efficient calorie burning. Innovative hydration methods, like tonic-infused electrolyte drinks, support hydration and nutrient balance during physical activities.

5.5 TAILORING FITNESS REGIMES FOR ENHANCED RESULTS WITH SUMATRA

Customizing fitness plans to include Sumatra Slim Belly Tonic can enhance workout performance and recovery. Whether starting with low-intensity exercises for beginners or incorporating high-intensity training for advanced athletes, the tonic supports muscle recovery and energy metabolism across fitness levels.

5.6 PSYCHOLOGICAL TECHNIQUES FOR SUSTAINED MOTIVATION

Addressing the psychological aspects of weight loss, such as motivation and goal setting, is vital. Sumatra Slim Belly Tonic can foster a positive mindset by improving physical well-being, which in turn reinforces motivation. Cognitive-behavioral techniques and celebrating successes can maintain long-term commitment, with the tonic serving as a reminder and enhancer of progress.

Buy Now

SUMATRA SLIM BELLY TONIC

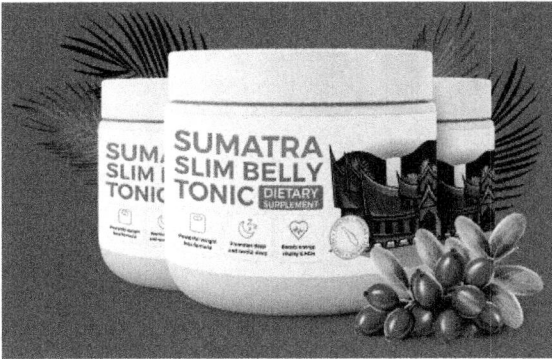

Is unlike anything you have ever seen or tried before It is the only product that contains a proprietary blend of 8 natural superfoods designed to rapidly target and optimize sleep quality. By fixing your interrupted and poor sleep your body will start to repair itself turning your body into a fat-burning furnace overnight

click the link or copy and past to your browser
https://e2a5f5kk0awwknchwegmy7j5a0.hop.clickbank.net

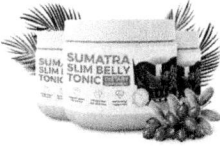

CHAPTER 6

Addressing Specific Health Concerns with Sumatra Slim Belly Tonic

I n this crucial chapter, we explore how Sumatra Slim Belly Tonic, with its robust blend of natural ingredients, stands not just as a supplement for general wellness but as a targeted therapeutic ally against specific health challenges. Here, we delve into the substantial benefits it offers to individuals battling diabetes—a condition that affects millions globally, disrupting lives with its complex metabolic implications.

6.1 SUMATRA SLIM BELLY TONIC FOR DIABETICS

Sumatra Slim Belly Tonic is a powerful ally for those managing diabetes, featuring Berberine, which enhances insulin sensitivity and stabilizes blood glucose levels by activating AMP-activated protein kinase (AMPK). This tonic also combats glycation, a process where excess sugar damages body tissues, thanks to antioxidants from Spirulina and Black Cohosh that inhibit harmful molecule formation. For optimal results, integrate this tonic with meals to support consistent blood sugar management.

Case Studies and Testimonials

John, a 58-year-old with type 2 diabetes, found significant blood sugar stabilization and increased energy after incorporating Sumatra Slim Belly Tonic into his routine. His experience, among others, showcases the tonic's transformative potential in diabetes care.

6.2 HEART HEALTH AND CHOLESTEROL MANAGEMENT WITH SUMATRA

Sumatra Slim Belly Tonic promotes cardiovascular health by managing blood lipid profiles and reducing arterial inflammation. Spirulina, a key ingredient, lowers LDL cholesterol and raises HDL cholesterol, mitigating the risk of heart attacks and strokes. Its anti-inflammatory properties ensure smooth blood flow and enhanced heart function. A heart-healthy diet alongside the tonic optimizes its benefits.

Success Stories

Sarah, a 45-year-old, saw a significant reduction in her cholesterol levels after adding the tonic to her regimen. Likewise, Mark, a 60-year-old with hypertension, experienced stabilized blood pressure and improved arterial health. These stories highlight the tonic's role in improving cardiovascular health.

As a working mother of three, finding time to take care of myself was always a challenge. But when I discovered Sumatra Slim Belly Tonic in just a few weeks, I've shed 26 pounds, I feel lighter on my feet and my joints feel supple... decades younger, my self-esteem is at an all time high too. I can't recommend it enough to anyone looking for a fast and effective weight loss solution, I feel amazing

— LAURA, 42 YEARS OLD

I've struggled with my weight for years, and body fat remove sumatra tonic has been a game-changer. The best part is that it helped improve my sleep quality, and I wake up feeling refreshed. The weight loss has been gradual but steady, and I've lost 15 pounds in just a couple of months. I highly recommend it!

— BEN THOMAS, 64 YEARS OLD

I never thought I would find a weight loss supplement that actually worked, but Sumatra Slim Belly Tonic has completely blown me away! I was initially skeptical, but this incredible product has exceeded all of my expectations. Not only has it helped me curb my cravings, but it has also improved my sleep quality. The best part? I have lost a whopping 20 pounds in just a few months! I couldn't be happier with the results. Thanks to Sumatra Slim Belly Tonic, I am finally on my way to achieving my dream body.

— ALEX S. - NEW YORK, USA

6.3 SUMATRA SLIM BELLY TONIC FOR POST-MENOPAUSAL WOMEN

This tonic offers relief from common menopausal symptoms like hot flashes and mood swings through ingredients like Black Cohosh and Humulus Lupulus. It supports bone health with nutrients essential for post-menopausal women, and aids in weight management by enhancing metabolic rate. Incorporating the tonic into a daily routine can help women navigate menopause more comfortably.

6.4 MANAGING THYROID ISSUES WITH SUMATRA

Sumatra Slim Belly Tonic supports thyroid health through Spirulina, which supplies iodine crucial for hormone production, and Ashwagandha, enhancing hormone secretion. It aids in weight management and energy stabilization for those with thyroid disorders. An integrative approach, combining the tonic with a diet rich in selenium and zinc and regular exercise, can amplify its effectiveness.

Precautionary Advice

Individuals with thyroid conditions should consult healthcare providers before starting any new supplement to avoid potential interactions with medications.

6.5 THE ROLE OF SUMATRA IN PREVENTING WEIGHT-RELATED JOINT PAIN

The tonic's anti-inflammatory ingredients, such as Inulin and Griffonia Simplicifolia, reduce joint pain and improve mobility. Its metabolism-boosting properties assist in effective weight management, lightening the load on stress-bearing joints. Nutritional support from Spirulina enhances joint health, making physical activities more manageable and enjoyable.

6.6 SUMATRA AND SKIN HEALTH: ACHIEVING A NATURAL GLOW

Sumatra Slim Belly Tonic detoxifies and nourishes the skin from within, thanks to ingredients like Inulin and Spirulina. Its antioxidants combat oxidative stress, slowing the aging process and enhancing skin vitality. Nutrients in the tonic support skin health, leading to a natural glow and improved complexion, as evidenced by users like Emily and David, who reported clearer, more vibrant skin.

SUMATRA SLIM BELLY TONIC

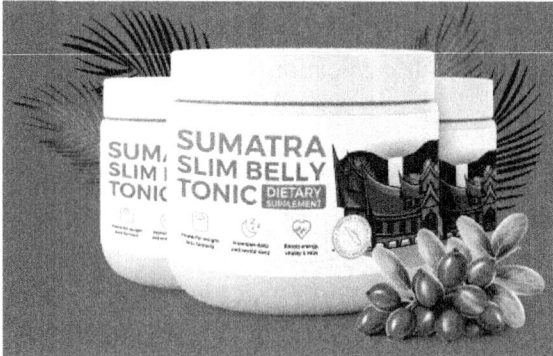

Is unlike anything you have ever seen or tried before It is the only product that contains a proprietary blend of 8 natural superfoods designed to rapidly target and optimize sleep quality. By fixing your interrupted and poor sleep your body will start to repair itself turning your body into a fat-burning furnace overnight

click the link or copy and past to your browser
https://e2a5f5kk0awwknchwegmy7j5a0.hop.clickbank.net

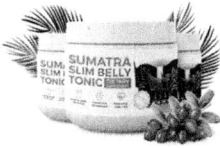

CHAPTER 7

The Psychological Journey of Weight Loss

W eight loss is as much a psychological endeavor as it is physical, intertwining the strength of the mind with the resilience of the body. As you embark on this transformative path with Sumatra Slim Belly Tonic at your side, understanding and overcoming the mental and emotional hurdles is crucial. This chapter delves into the foundational aspect of building psychological resilience against the inevitable setbacks that accompany the journey of weight loss, ensuring you are equipped not only to face these challenges but to emerge stronger from them.

7.1 BUILDING RESILIENCE AGAINST WEIGHT LOSS SETBACKS

Understanding Setbacks as Part of the Journey

Setbacks such as stagnant weight, overwhelming cravings, or disrupted workout plans are not failures but essential learning moments in your weight loss journey. They offer insights into your dietary habits, bodily responses, and emotional triggers. Embracing setbacks as natural allows you to navigate the weight loss process with resilience, preparing you for a journey filled with both challenges and triumphs.

Strategies for Building Resilience

Resilience is key to weight loss, fostered by setting realistic goals and celebrating every success, no matter how small. Incorporating Sumatra Slim Belly Tonic into your daily regimen can support metabolic resilience and act as a tangible step toward achieving your overall health goals. Adaptability, such as modifying exercise routines or choosing healthy food alternatives, further strengthens resilience.

Learning from Setbacks

Each setback is an opportunity to identify and understand patterns or triggers that may impede progress. Recognizing stress or a lack of preparation as triggers allows for the development of effective coping strategies, like integrating stress-management techniques or proactive meal planning.

Role of Support Systems

A strong support network provides both emotional and practical support, offering encouragement, sharing healthy living tips, and understanding your weight loss goals. Regular engagement with supportive friends, family, or groups reinforces your commitment and motivates you through challenges.

7.2 THE ROLE OF POSITIVE SELF-TALK IN WEIGHT MANAGEMENT

Transforming negative self-talk into positive affirmations is vital. Replacing detrimental thoughts with messages of strength and possibility promotes a supportive mindset, essential for a successful weight loss journey. Practices like gratitude journaling and repeating positive mantras can solidify this positive mindset.

7.3 VISUALIZATION TECHNIQUES FOR ACHIEVING YOUR IDEAL WEIGHT

Visualization involves creating a detailed mental image of reaching your weight loss goals, incorporating associated emotions and experiences. This powerful technique can motivate action and foster a positive mindset by vividly imagining success and the steps needed to achieve it.

7.4 HOW TO USE JOURNALING FOR WEIGHT LOSS SUCCESS

Journaling offers a reflective insight into your personal health journey, documenting emotions, dietary habits, and physical activities. It encourages mindfulness, aids in stress management, and tracks progress, serving as a transformative tool for personal growth and weight loss success.

7.5 THE CONNECTION BETWEEN BODY IMAGE AND WEIGHT SUCCESS

A positive body image supports healthy behaviors and self-care, while a negative image can promote harmful habits. Improving body image involves focusing on functional goals and appreciating your body's capabilities, countering the unrealistic standards often depicted in media.

7.6 OVERCOMING THE FEAR OF SUCCESS IN WEIGHT LOSS

The fear of success, manifesting as self-sabotage or anxiety over changes, can impede weight loss efforts. Addressing this fear through cognitive-behavioral techniques, affirmations, and professional support can pave the way for a successful and transformative journey. Achieving weight loss is more than physical transformation; it's about overcoming psychological barriers and fostering a positive, resilient mindset. This chapter equips you with strategies to navigate these challenges, supporting a sustainable and successful weight loss journey.

Buy Now

SUMATRA SLIM BELLY TONIC

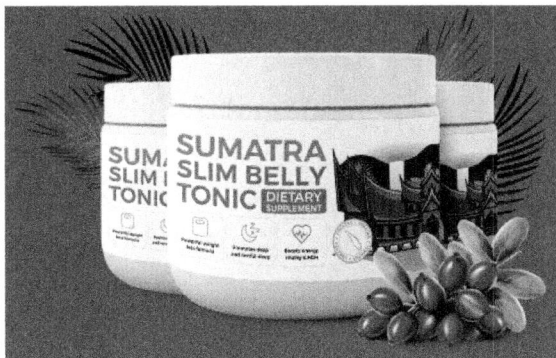

Is unlike anything you have ever seen or tried before It is the only product that contains a proprietary blend of 8 natural superfoods designed to rapidly target and optimize sleep quality. By fixing your interrupted and poor sleep your body will start to repair itself turning your body into a fat-burning furnace overnight

click the link or copy and past to your browser
https://e2a5f5kk0awwknchwegmy7j5a0.hop.clickbank.net

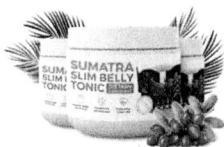

CHAPTER 8

Beyond the Scale

GAUGING YOUR SUCCESS

I n a world obsessed with scale victories, it's essential to understand and embrace the broader spectrum of health indicators. Weight loss, while significant, is only one facet of a multifaceted journey toward wellness. This chapter, "Beyond the Scale," invites you to explore the deeper, often overlooked aspects of health transformation, particularly focusing on body composition changes—a critical but less visible aspect of your health improvement journey.

8.1 UNDERSTANDING AND MEASURING BODY COMPOSITION CHANGES

Explaining Body Composition

Understanding body composition is essential for anyone embarking on a health journey with Sumatra Slim Belly Tonic. It offers a detailed view of health, revealing the ratios of fat, muscle, bone, and water in the body. This perspective moves beyond mere weight to assess the balance of lean mass to fat, providing a more accurate reflection of health and progress.

Tools for Measuring Body Composition

Tools like the Dual-Energy X-ray Absorptiometry (DEXA) scans offer precise body composition analysis, but more accessible methods such as bioelectrical impedance analysis (BIA) and skinfold measurements with calipers can also provide valuable insights into your body's makeup and changes over time.

Interpreting Results

Results from body composition measurements can guide your health regimen adjustments, informing dietary, exercise, and Sumatra Slim Belly Tonic intake to optimize outcomes. Positive changes in body composition, such as a reduction in fat mass and an increase in muscle mass, underscore the effectiveness of your efforts beyond what the scale shows.

Impact of Sumatra Slim Belly Tonic on Body Composition

Sumatra Slim Belly Tonic supports the transformation of body composition by enhancing metabolic health and aiding in fat reduction while encouraging muscle preservation and growth. Ingredients like Spirulina and Berberine play key roles in improving endurance, strength, and metabolism, fostering a physique that's not only leaner but healthier and more resilient.

8.2 THE IMPORTANCE OF NON-SCALE VICTORIES

Non-Scale Victories (NSVs) are critical markers of progress, including increased energy, better-fitting clothes, and improvements in health markers like blood pressure or blood sugar levels. Documenting and celebrating these victories can significantly boost motivation and provide a more comprehensive view of health improvements. Sumatra Slim Belly Tonic contributes to various NSVs, such as enhanced energy levels and improved physical comfort, due to its metabolism-boosting and anti-inflammatory properties. Recognizing these victories underscores the tonic's role in achieving a more vibrant and active lifestyle.

8.3 HOW TO MAINTAIN WEIGHT LOSS WITH SUMATRA SLIM BELLY TONIC

Maintaining weight loss involves a permanent lifestyle change, where Sumatra Slim Belly Tonic continues to play a vital role by stabilizing metabolism and reducing cravings. Adjusting dosage and integrating the tonic into a balanced lifestyle that includes regular physical activity and nutrition is key to sustaining weight management efforts.

8.4 CELEBRATING MILESTONES AND SETTING NEW HEALTH GOALS

Celebrating milestones and setting new health and wellness goals are essential for continued motivation and progress. Incorporating Sumatra Slim Belly Tonic into these goals supports nutritional needs and adapts to changing health objectives, whether they involve increased physical activity or a focus on other aspects of health.

8.5 THE ROLE OF COMMUNITY SUPPORT IN MAINTAINING WEIGHT LOSS

Community support is invaluable in the weight loss journey, providing motivation, accountability, and shared knowledge. Engaging with supportive groups, participating in discussions, and organizing activities around Sumatra Slim Belly Tonic can enhance commitment and enrich the journey with shared experiences and triumphs.

8.6 REFLECTING ON YOUR JOURNEY AND PLANNING FOR THE FUTURE

Reflecting on your journey helps to appreciate the transformation and to learn from it, informing future health plans. As you set new goals, consider how Sumatra Slim Belly Tonic can continue to support your health, adapting its use to align with evolving needs and objectives. This ongoing engagement with your health, supported by the tonic, ensures a dynamic approach to wellness that fosters continual growth and vitality.

Buy Now

SUMATRA SLIM BELLY TONIC

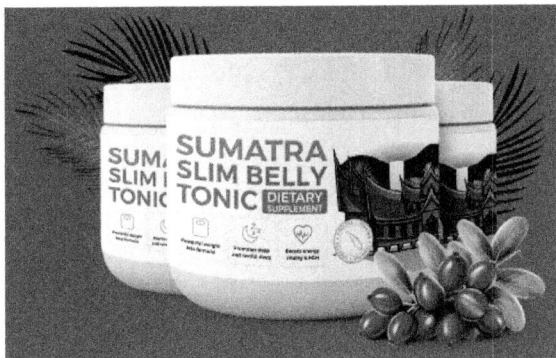

Is unlike anything you have ever seen or tried before It is the only product that contains a proprietary blend of 8 natural superfoods designed to rapidly target and optimize sleep quality. By fixing your interrupted and poor sleep your body will start to repair itself turning your body into a fat-burning furnace overnight

click the link or copy and past to your browser
https://e2a5f5kk0awwknchwegmy7j5a0.hop.clickbank.net

Share Your Success and Keep the Momentum Going

Think how much you have changed, physically and mentally. You are starting to feel more confident in your body and thriving in the new lifestyle. It's an incredible gift to be able to pass this on to someone else.

LEAVE A REVIEW!

Just a few minutes of your time can transform the next person's life. In advance, thank you and I am extremely grateful. I can't wait to hear about your personal journeys, so good luck and keep up the good work so those results keep shining!

Scan the QR code below or follow this link:
https://www.amazon.com/review/create-review/?
asin=B0DFB733WY

Conclusion

As we reach the conclusion of our journey together through "Natural Health Weight Loss with Sumatra Slim Belly Tonic," it's important to reflect on the transformative path we've embarked upon. From understanding the science behind the potent Sumatra Slim Belly Tonic, navigating through comprehensive dietary guidelines, to tackling specific health concerns and the psychological facets of weight loss, this journey has been about much more than shedding pounds. It has been about embracing a holistic approach to wellness that integrates not just our physical health, but our mental and emotional well-being too.

Sumatra Slim Belly Tonic is not just a supplement; it's a catalyst for change. Its carefully selected organic ingredients boost metabolism, enhance mood, improve sleep quality, and promote fat burning. More importantly, they support a spectrum of health benefits—from improving gut health and balancing hormones to reducing inflammation and enhancing skin health. This tonic is designed to be a part of a lifestyle shift that encourages a comprehensive approach to health and well-being.

However, achieving and maintaining weight loss is more than about what we consume; it's about transforming our lifestyle. Sustainable changes—integrating healthy eating, regular physical activities, and mindfulness practices—are crucial. It's these changes that will carry us forward to a healthier life, not just in the short run but as a permanent way of living.

The role of community and the support of like-minded individuals cannot be overstressed. Whether it's family, friends, or online communities, having a support network provides motivation, accountability, and the sharing of invaluable insights and encouragement. I urge you to reach out, connect, and even share your own stories of transformation. In doing so, you strengthen not only your own resolve but also inspire others on their paths.

Now, as you stand at the threshold of this journey, I encourage you to take that first step. Begin with introducing Sumatra Slim Belly Tonic into your daily routine, but remember, this journey extends beyond the physical aspects of weight loss. It's about cultivating a vibrant, healthier life full of energy and wellness.

Continue to educate yourself, remain adaptable, and be responsive to your body's needs. Health and well-being are dynamic; they evolve as we do, and staying informed and flexible is key to sustaining success. Share your progress, celebrate your successes, and never hesitate to seek guidance and support.

In closing, I leave you with a message of hope and empowerment. Each one of you has the innate strength and the capability to transform your health and your life. With Sumatra Slim Belly Tonic as a part of your arsenal and this book as your guide, you are well-equipped to embark on this rewarding path. Remember, every journey begins with a single step, and every day presents a new opportunity to move closer to your health and wellness goals.

Together, let's embrace these possibilities and make the most of the vibrant health and vitality that awaits us. Here's to a healthier, happier you!

References

- *Sumatra Slim Belly Tonic Reviews Supplement Does it ...* https:// bentleysystems.service-now.com/community?id= community_question&sys_id=0fc56a0687130e10416d cbb7dabb350f
- *Therapeutic effect of berberine on metabolic diseases* https://www. sciencedirect.com/science/article/pii/S0753332220311768
- *The effects of a thermogenic supplement on metabolic and ...* https://www.ncbi.nlm.nih.gov/pmc/articles/PMC9987759/
- *A Systematic Review of Dietary Supplements and ...* https://www. ncbi.nlm.nih.gov/pmc/articles/PMC8231729/
- *Sumatra Slim Belly Tonic Pro Review - What is This 7 ...* https:// www.bellevuereporter.com/wellness/sumatra-slim-belly-tonic-pro-review-what-is-this-7-second-bedtime-hack-everyone-is-talking-about/
- *Healthy meals start with planning* https://www.mayoclinic.org/ healthy-lifestyle/nutrition-and-healthy-eating/in-depth/healthy-meals/art-20546806
- *31 Healthy Metabolism-Boosting Recipes - Eat This Not That* https://www.eatthis.com/metabolism-boosting-recipes-weight-loss/
- *Nutrient Timing: What to Eat Before and After a Workout* https:// blog.nasm.org/workout-and-nutrition-timing
- *Getting past a weight-loss plateau* https://www.mayoclinic.org/ healthy-lifestyle/weight-loss/in-depth/weight-loss-plateau/art-20044615
- *12 Effective Ways to Cope with Drug and Alcohol Cravings* https:// recoverycovepa.com/blog/12-effective-ways-cope-drug-alcohol-cravings/
- *Berberine: A Powerful Supplement with Many Benefits* https:// www.healthline.com/nutrition/berberine-powerful-supplement
- *Sumatra Slim Belly Tonic Review - Does This 7 Second ...* https:// www.covingtonreporter.com/life/sumatra-slim-belly-tonic-review-does-this-7-second-bedtime-hack-really-work/

- *Sleep and Metabolism: An Overview - PMC* https://www.ncbi.nlm. nih.gov/pmc/articles/PMC2929498/
- *How Stress Can Lead to Weight Gain, and How to Fight It* https:// www.everydayhealth.com/wellness/united-states-of-stress/how-stress-can-lead-weight-gain-how-fight-it/
- *Mindful Eating: The Art of Presence While You Eat - PMC* https:// www.ncbi.nlm.nih.gov/pmc/articles/PMC5556586/
- *The 9 Best Diet Plans: Sustainability, Weight Loss, and More* https://www.healthline.com/nutrition/best-diet-plans
- *Intermittent Fasting: Benefits, Side Effects, Quality of Life, ...* https://www.ncbi.nlm.nih.gov/pmc/articles/PMC9998115/
- *The Best Macronutrient Ratio for Weight Loss* https://www. healthline.com/nutrition/best-macronutrient-ratio
- *Food synergy: an operational concept for understanding ...* https:// www.ncbi.nlm.nih.gov/pmc/articles/PMC2731586/
- *Motivation, self-determination, and long-term weight control* https://www.ncbi.nlm.nih.gov/pmc/articles/PMC3312817/
- *Effects of berberine on glucose-lipid metabolism ...* https://www. ncbi.nlm.nih.gov/pmc/articles/PMC6434235/
- *Effects of spirulina on weight loss and blood lipids: a review* https://openheart.bmj.com/content/7/1/e001003
- *Weight gain during the menopause transition: Evidence for a ...* https://obgyn.onlinelibrary.wiley.com/doi/10.1111/1471-0528. 17290
- *8 Natural Supplements That Help Fight Inflammation* https://www. medicalnewstoday.com/articles/326067
- *How losing weight can impact mental health* https://www.healio. com/news/primary-care/20230622/mental-health-and-weight-loss-how-losing-weight-can-impact-mental-health
- *Resilience in weight management – Metamed* https://metamed.ca/ resilience-in-weight-management/
- *The power of positive self-talk in weight loss success* https://www. hypnotherapy-directory.org.uk/memberarticles/the-power-of-positive-self-talk-in-weight-loss-success
- *How Visualization Can Benefit Your Well-Being* https://www. psychologytoday.com/us/blog/click-here-for-happiness/202308/ how-visualization-can-benefit-your-well-being
- *Body fat scale accuracy: How they work and alternative methods*

https://www.medicalnewstoday.com/articles/body-fat-scale-accuracy

- *15 Non-Scale Victories to Celebrate for Weight Loss* https://www.healthline.com/health/non-scale-victories
- *The 17 Best Ways to Maintain Weight Loss* https://www.healthline.com/nutrition/maintain-weight-loss
- *Sumatra Slim Belly Tonic Review: My 5-Month Experience* https://mdtheatreguide.com/shows/sumatra-slim-belly-tonic-review-my-5-month-experience/
- Lunders, Katelyn, Lauren Smith McDonough, and Corinne Sullivan. 2024. "20 weight loss motivation quotes that'll empower you to keep going." *Woman's Day*, July 31, 2024. https://www.womansday.com/health-fitness/womens-health/g3209/best-weight-loss-motivation/

Printed in Great Britain
by Amazon

60577139R00047